Travell, Simons & Simons' Trigger Point Pain Patterns

FLIP CHARTS

Second Edition

Anatomical Chart Company

Contributing Consultant:

Joseph M. Donnelly, PT, DHS, OCS

Travell, Simons & Simons' Trigger Point Pain Patterns Flip Charts are organized in six sections following the structure of the Clinical Considerations chapters in *Travell, Simons & Simons' Myofascial Pain and Dysfunction: The Trigger Point Manual,* Third Edition. Each section contains Trigger Point (TrP) pain referral patterns that may cause or be associated with a clinical condition commonly seen in clinical practice. The selection of TrP referral patterns is based on research and those identified in the Clinical Considerations chapters. The organization of the flip charts is intended to be a quick clinical reference to include TrPs as part of the clinical examination. The clinician should palpate the entire muscle from origin to insertion using cross-fiber flat or pincer palpation to identify the most painful spot (TrP) in the taut band.

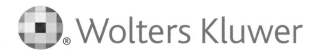. Wolters Kluwer

Philadelphia • Baltimore • New York • London
Buenos Aires • Hong Kong • Sydney • Tokyo

Acquisitions Editor: Crystal Taylor
Senior Development Editor: Amy Millholen
Production Project Manager: Justin Wright
Marketing Manager: Phyllis Hitner
Manager, Graphic Arts & Design: Stephen Druding
Manufacturing Coordinator: Beth Welsh
Prepress Vendor: Straive

9 8 7 6 5 4 3 2 1
Printed in China

Cataloging-in-Publication Data available on request from the Publisher
ISBN: 978-1-9751-8378-3

This work is provided "as is," and the publisher disclaims any and all warranties, express or implied, including any warranties as to accuracy, comprehensiveness, or currency of the content of this work.

This work is no substitute for individual patient assessment based upon healthcare professionals' examination of each patient and consideration of, among other things, age, weight, gender, current or prior medical conditions, medication history, laboratory data and other factors unique to the patient. The publisher does not provide medical advice or guidance and this work is merely a reference tool. Healthcare professionals, and not the publisher, are solely responsible for the use of this work including all medical judgments and for any resulting diagnosis and treatments.

Given continuous, rapid advances in medical science and health information, independent professional verification of medical diagnoses, indications, appropriate pharmaceutical selections and dosages, and treatment options should be made and healthcare professionals should consult a variety of sources. When prescribing medication, healthcare professionals are advised to consult the product information sheet (the manufacturer's package insert) accompanying each drug to verify, among other things, conditions of use, warnings and side effects and identify any changes in dosage schedule or contraindications, particularly if the medication to be administered is new, infrequently used or has a narrow therapeutic range. To the maximum extent permitted under applicable law, no responsibility is assumed by the publisher for any injury and/or damage to persons or property, as a matter of products liability, negligence law or otherwise, or from any reference to or use by any person of this work.

shop.lww.com

TABLE OF CONTENTS

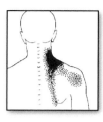
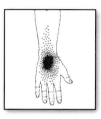
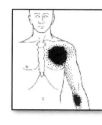
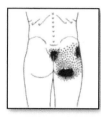
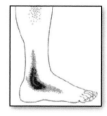

Tension-Type Headache

Chapter 18

Upper trapezius

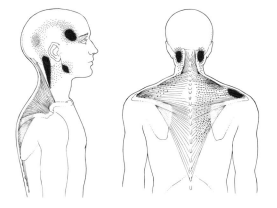

Sternocleidomastoid

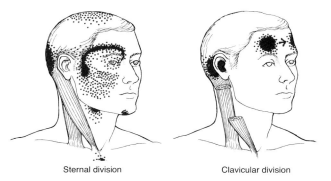

Sternal division   Clavicular division

Masseter

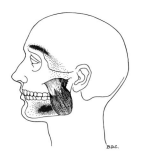

Suboccipital

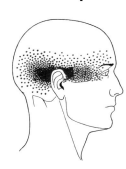

Temporalis

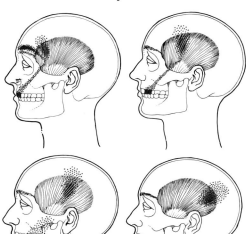

Splenius cervicis

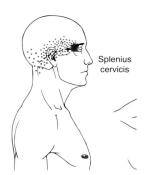

Splenius cervicis

Semispinalis capitis

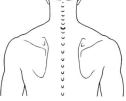

Cervicogenic Headache (Unilateral)

Chapter 18

Upper trapezius

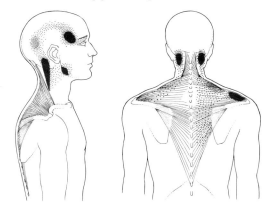

Sternocleidomastoid

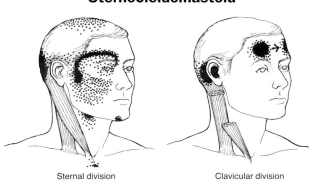

Sternal division   Clavicular division

Suboccipital

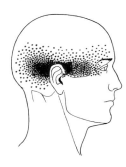

Splenius cervicis

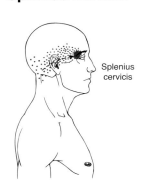

Splenius cervicis

Semispinalis capitis

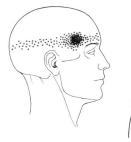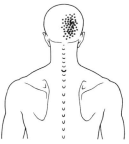

Migraine Headache

Upper trapezius
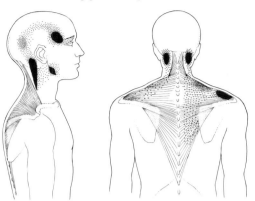

Sternocleidomastoid
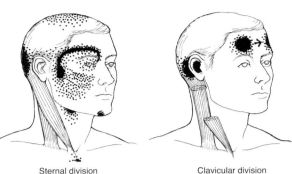
Sternal division
Clavicular division

Temporalis
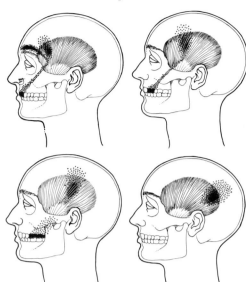

TMJ (Jaw and Tooth Pain)

Temporalis
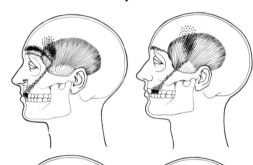

Medial pterygoid
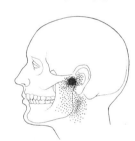
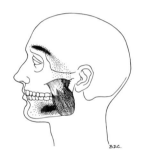

Masseter
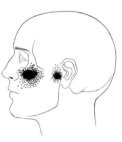

Lateral pterygoid
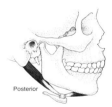

Anterior and posterior digastric
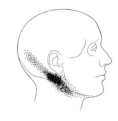
Posterior
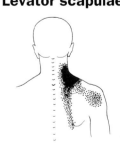
Anterior

Neck Pain

Upper trapezius
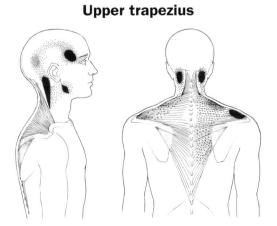

Splenius cervicis
Splenius cervicis
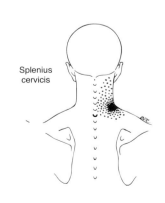

Posterior cervical
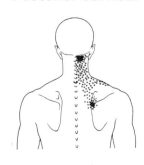

Levator scapulae

Infraspinatus
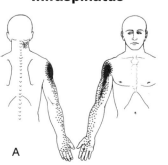
A

Scalenes   **Supraspinatus**   **Infraspinatus**   **Deltoid**   **Pectoralis minor**

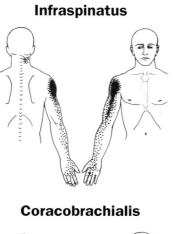

Coracobrachialis   **Biceps brachii**

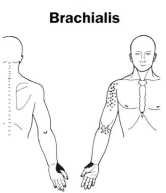

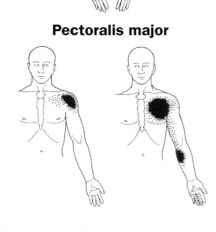

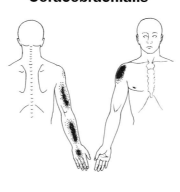

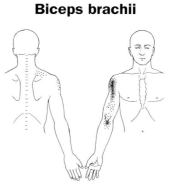

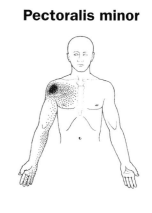

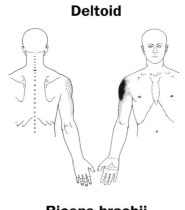

Brachialis   **Pectoralis major**

Teres minor   **Latissimus dorsi**   **Teres major**   **Subscapularis**   **Deltoid**

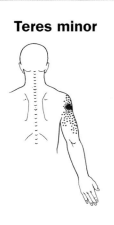

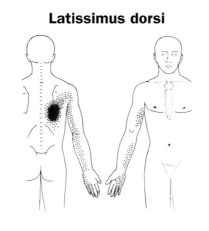

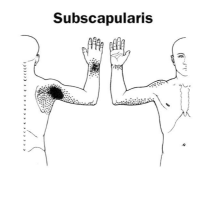

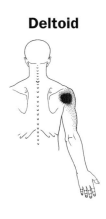

Triceps brachii   **Levator scapulae**

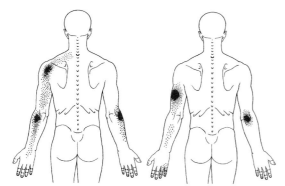

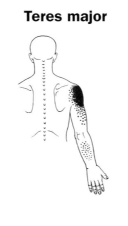

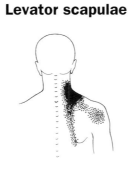

Thoracic Outlet Syndrome

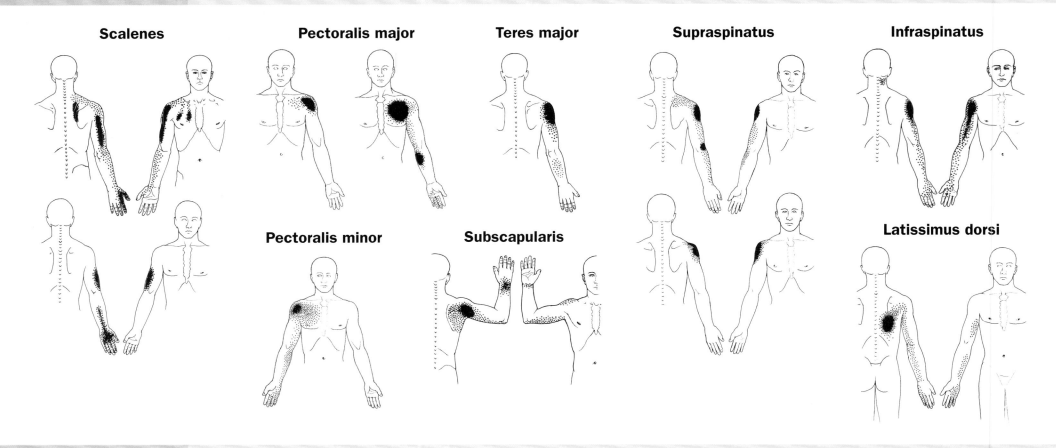

Scalenes

Pectoralis major

Teres major

Supraspinatus

Infraspinatus

Pectoralis minor

Subscapularis

Latissimus dorsi

Subacromial Pain Syndrome

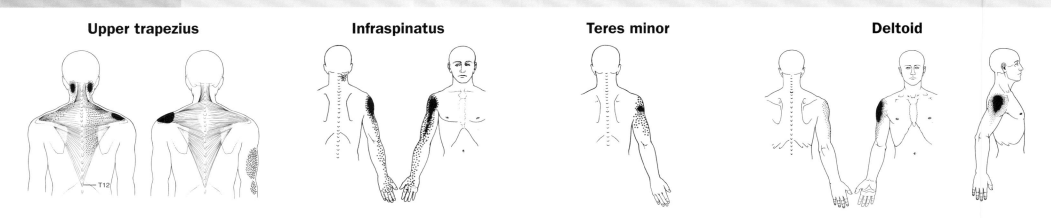

Upper trapezius

Infraspinatus

Teres minor

Deltoid

Shoulder Impingement Syndrome

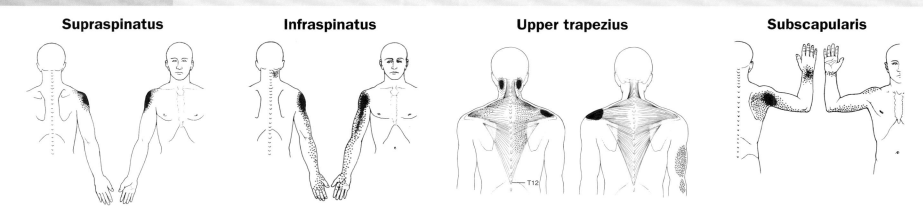

Supraspinatus

Infraspinatus

Upper trapezius

Subscapularis

Frozen Shoulder (Adhesive Capsulitis) Chapter 33

Subscapularis

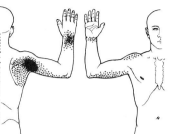

Infraspinatus

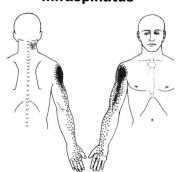

Supraspinatus

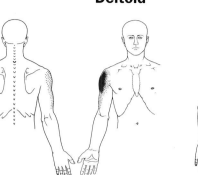

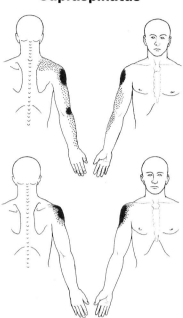

Deltoid

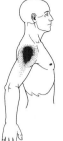

Medial Border of Scapula Pain (Shoulder Blade) Chapter 33

Levator scapulae

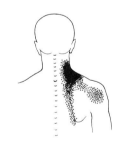

Scalenes

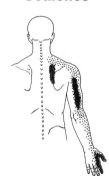

Infraspinatus

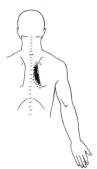

Latissimus dorsi

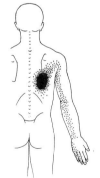

Serratus anterior

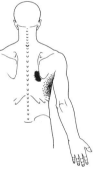

Middle trapezius

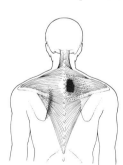

Iliocostalis thoracis

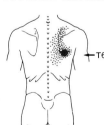

Serratus posterior superior

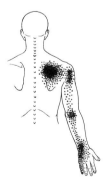

Thoracic multifidi

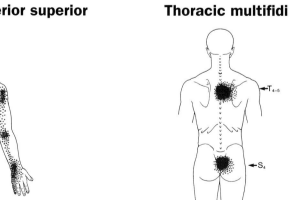

Rhomboid

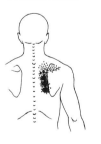

Lateral Epicondylalgia (Tennis Elbow)

Chapter 41

Supraspinatus **Supinator** **Triceps brachii** **Anconeus**

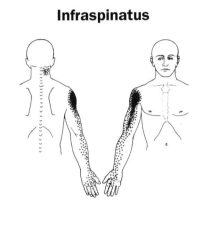

Lateral Epicondylalgia with Forearm Pain
Chapter 41

Infraspinatus **Extensor carpi ulnaris** **Extensor carpi radialis brevis** **Extensor digitorum**

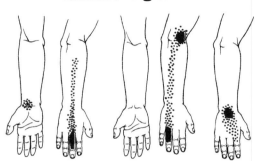

Extensor carpi radialis longus **Brachioradialis**

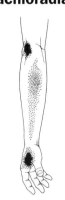

Medial Epicondylalgia (Golfer's Elbow)
Chapter 41

Pronator teres **Pronator quadratus** **Pectoralis major** **Latissimus dorsi** **Subscapularis**

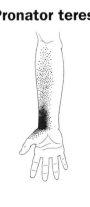
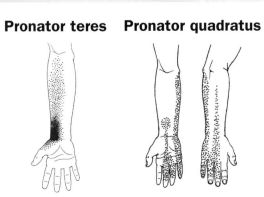
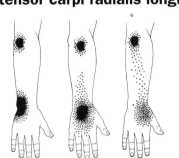
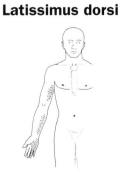
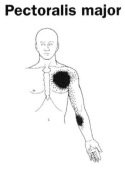
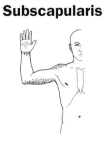

Radial Forearm, Wrist, and Thumb Pain

Pronator teres

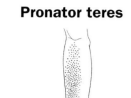

Brachialis

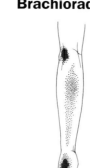

Supinator

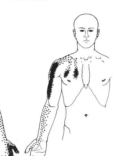

Brachioradialis

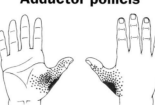

Extensor carpi radialis longus

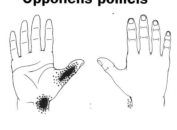

Infraspinatus

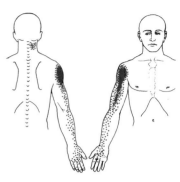

Scalenii

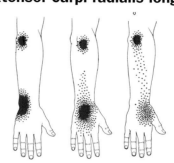

Adductor pollicis

Opponens pollicis

Ulnar Forearm and Wrist Pain

Latissimus dorsi

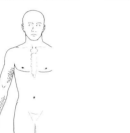

Extensor carpi ulnaris

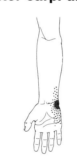

Flexor carpi ulnaris

Flexor digitorum superficialis and profundus

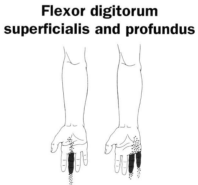

Pronator quadratus

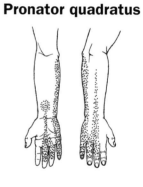

Dorsal Forearm and Wrist Pain

Subscapularis

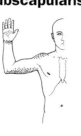

Teres major

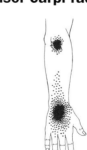

Extensor carpi radialis brevis

Extensor indicis

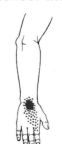

Finger and Hand Pain

Chapter 41

Flexor digitorum superficialis and profundus

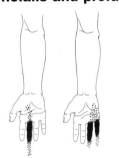

Flexor pollicis longus

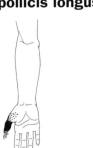

Pronator quadratus

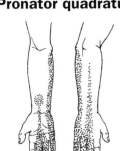

Extensor digitorum

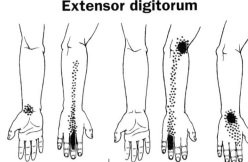

Palmaris longus

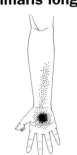

Carpal Tunnel Syndrome

Chapter 41

Infraspinatus

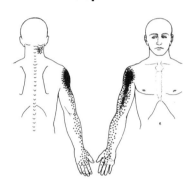

Subscapularis

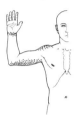

Pronator teres

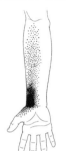

Flexor carpi radialis

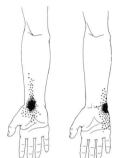

Palmaris longus

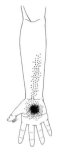

8

Low Back Pain

Composite

Iliocostalis Lumborum
Multifidus - L2, S 1
Iliopsoas

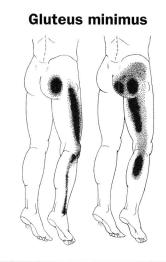

Gluteus medius

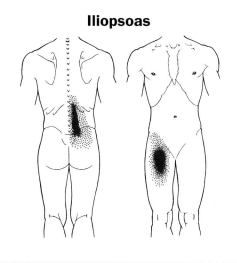

Rectus abdominus

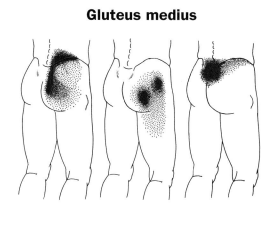

Low Back Pain with Leg Pain

Piriformis
Gluteus minimus
Iliopsoas
Tensor fascia latae
Gluteus medius

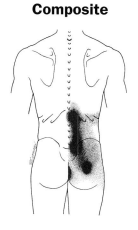
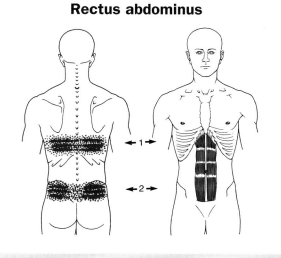
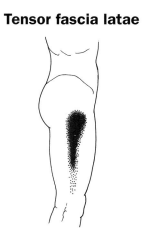

Low Back Pain with Buttock Pain

Iliocostalis lumborum
Longissimus thoracis
Deep paraspinals

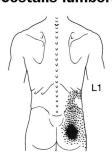
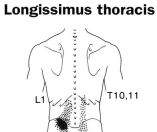
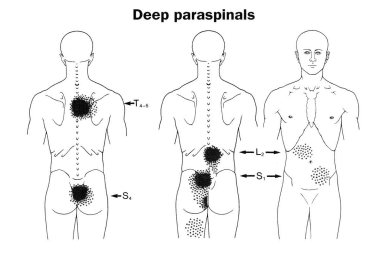

9

Post Lumbar Laminectomy Syndrome Chapter 53

Quadratus lumborum

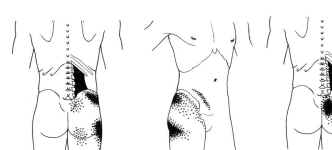

Gluteus medius

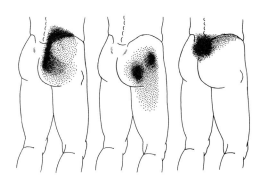

Iliocostalis lumborum

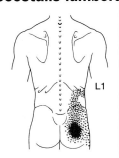

Sacroiliac Joint and Buttock Pain Chapter 53

Composite
Quadratus lumborum
Levator Ani
Gluteus maximus
Puriformis

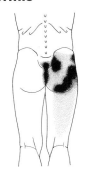

Quadratus lumborum

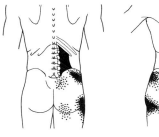

Piriformis

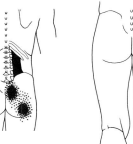

Gluteus minimus

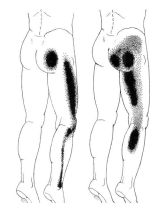

Gluteus medius

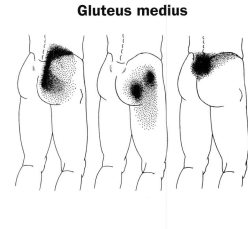

Multifidus

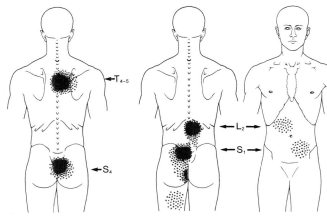

Thoracolumbar paraspinals

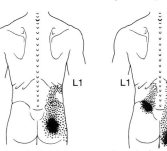

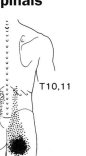

Gluteus maximus

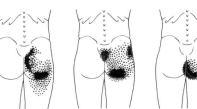

Levator Ani

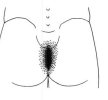

Levator ani

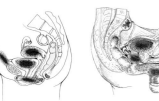

External abdominal oblique

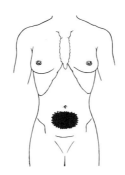

Rectus abdominus

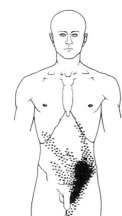

Adductor magnus

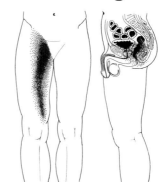

Gluteus medius

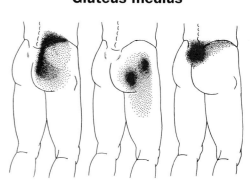

Pubococcygeus

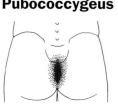

Levator ani

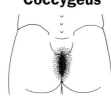

Coccygeus

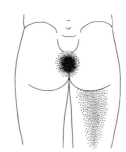

Obturator internus

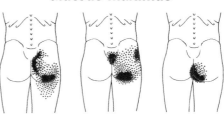

Gluteus maximus

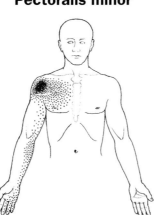 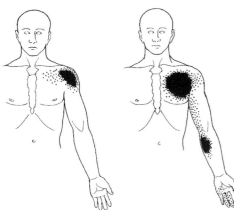 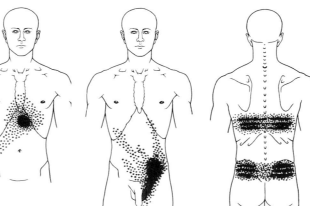

Pectoralis major

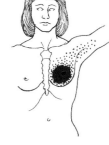 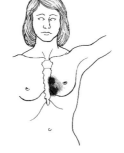

Pectoralis minor

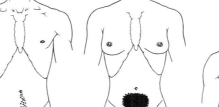 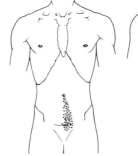

Abdominal muscles

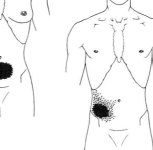 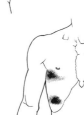

Iliocostalis thoracis

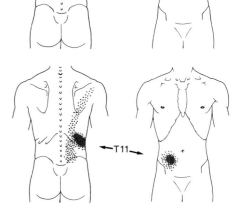

Diaphragm

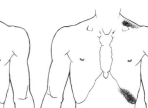

Hip Osteoarthritis

Gluteus medius   **Gluteus minimus**   **Tensor fascia latae**   **Pectineus**   **Adductor longus/brevis**   **Piriformis**

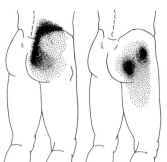 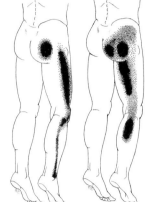 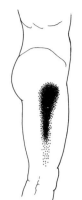 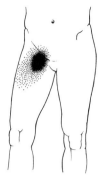 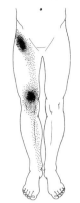 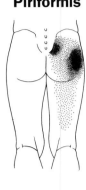

Femoral Acetabular Impingement/
Labral Tear/Athletic Pubalgia (Groin Pain)

Iliopsoas   **Tensor fascia latae**   **Rectus abdominus**   **External abdominal oblique**   **Adductor longus/brevis**   **Pectineus**

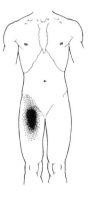 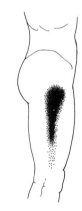 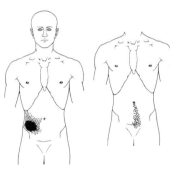 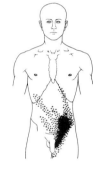 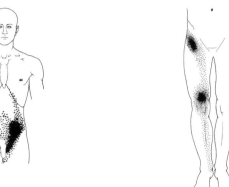 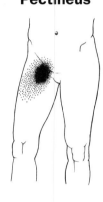

Greater Trochanteric Pain Syndrome

Tensor fascia latae   **Vastus lateralis**   **Gluteus maximus**   **Gluteus medius**   **Gluteus minimus**   **Quadratus lumborum**

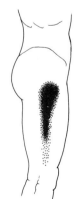 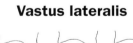 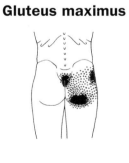 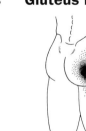 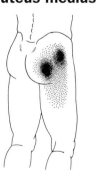 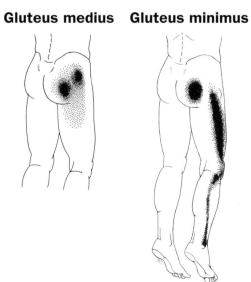 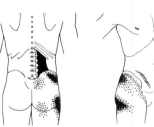

5 HIP, THIGH, AND KNEE PAIN

Piriformis Syndrome

Chapter 62

Piriformis	Semimembranosus/Semitendonosis	Gluteus maximus	Gluteus medius	Gluteus minimus	Quadratus lumborum

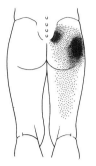 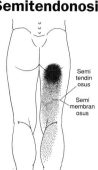 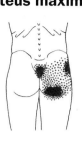 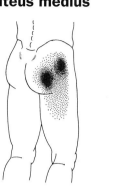 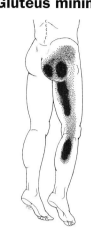 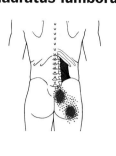

Patellofemoral Pain Syndrome

Chapter 62

Rectus femoris	Vastus lateralis	Vastus medialis	Vastus intermedius	Adductor longus/brevis

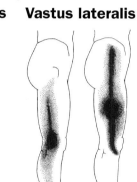 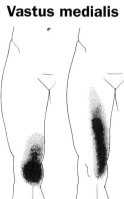 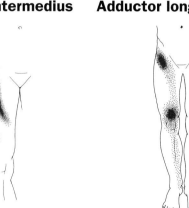 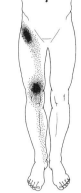

Knee Osteoarthritis

Chapter 62

Rectus femoris	Vastus lateralis	Vastus medialis	Vastus intermedius	Adductor magnus	Adductor longus/brevis

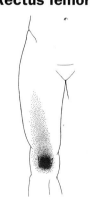 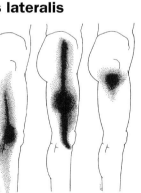 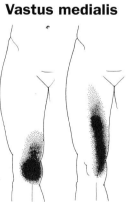 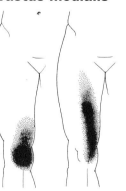 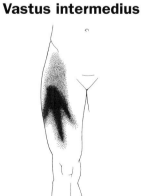 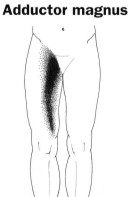 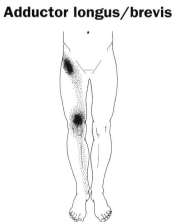

Gracilis	Biceps femoris	Semitendinosus/semimembranosus	Gastrocnemius	Popliteus

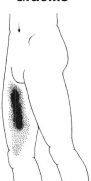 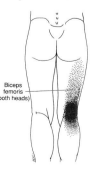 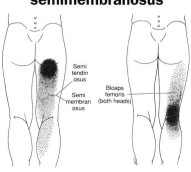 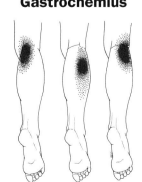 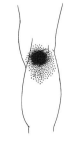

Iliotibial Band Syndrome Chapter 62

Vastus lateralis

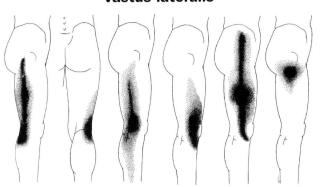

Tensor fascia latae

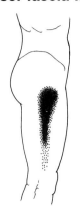

Gluteus medius

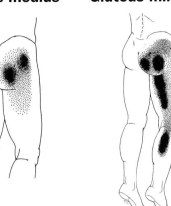

Gluteus minimus

Posterior Thigh and Knee Pain Chapter 62

Hamstring muscles

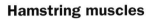
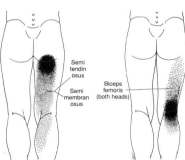

Semi tendin osus

Semi membran osus

Biceps femoris (both heads)

Gastrocnemius

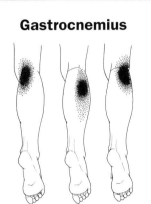

Soleus

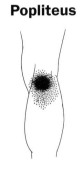

Popliteus

Knee Injuries (Ligaments, Meniscus) Chapter 62

Rectus femoris

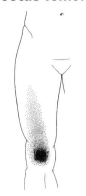

Vastus lateralis

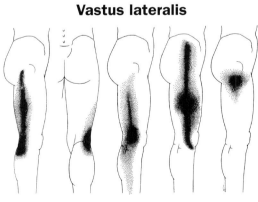

Vastus medialis

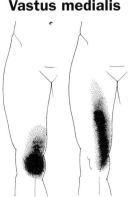

Sartorius

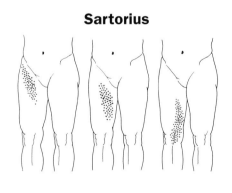

Adductor longus/brevis

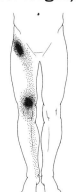

Gracilis

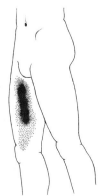

6 LEG, ANKLE, AND FOOT PAIN

Lateral Ankle Sprain/Instability   Chapter 71

Fibularis longus/brevis

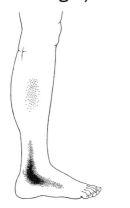

Fibularis tertius

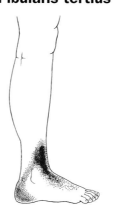

Tibialis anterior

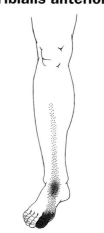

Nocturnal Calf Cramps   Chapter 71

Gastrocnemius

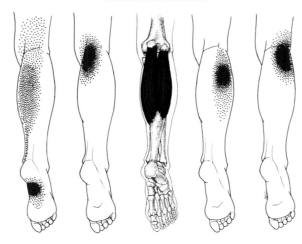

Dorsal Ankle and Foot Pain   Chapter 71

Tibialis anterior

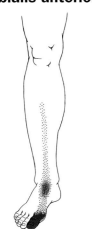

Fibularis tertius

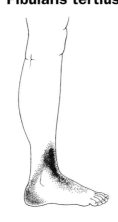

Extensor digitorum longus

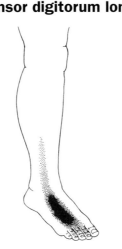

Extensor hallucis longus

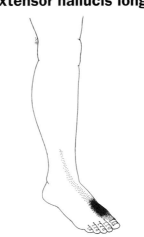

Extensor digitorum/hallucis brevis

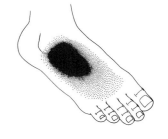

Achilles Tendon Pain

Soleus

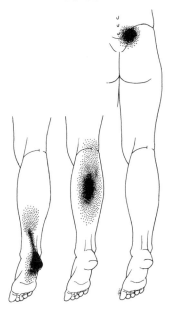

Gastrocnemius

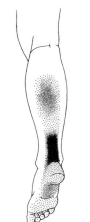

Tibialis posterior

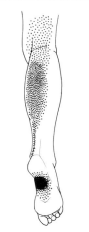

Abductor hallucis

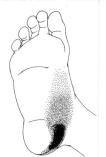

Tarsal Tunnel Syndrome

Flexor digitorum longus

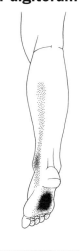

Abductor hallucis

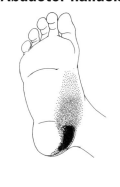

Flexor accessorius (quadratus plantae)

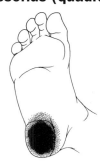

Plantar Foot/Heel Pain
(Plantar Fascialgia, Plantar Fasciitis)

Gastrocnemius

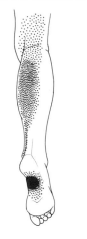

Soleus

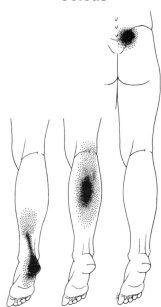

Tibialis posterior

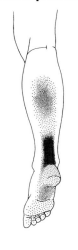

Flexor digitorum longus

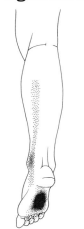

Flexor accessorius (quadratus plantae)

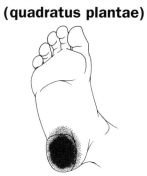

Abductor hallucis

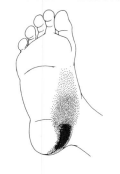

6 LEG, ANKLE, AND FOOT PAIN

Metatarsalgia (Ball of Foot Pain)   Chapter 71

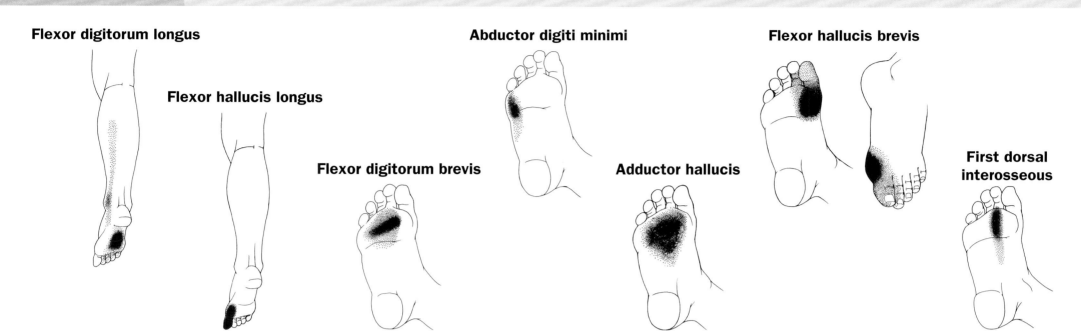

Flexor digitorum longus

Flexor hallucis longus

Flexor digitorum brevis

Abductor digiti minimi

Adductor hallucis

Flexor hallucis brevis

First dorsal interosseous

Hallux Valgus/Great Toe Pain/Sesamoiditis   Chapter 71

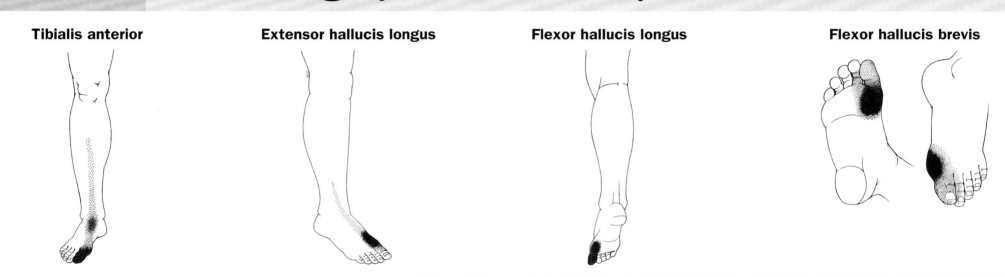

Tibialis anterior

Extensor hallucis longus

Flexor hallucis longus

Flexor hallucis brevis

Morton's Neuroma/Intertarsal Pain/Toe Pain   Chapter 71

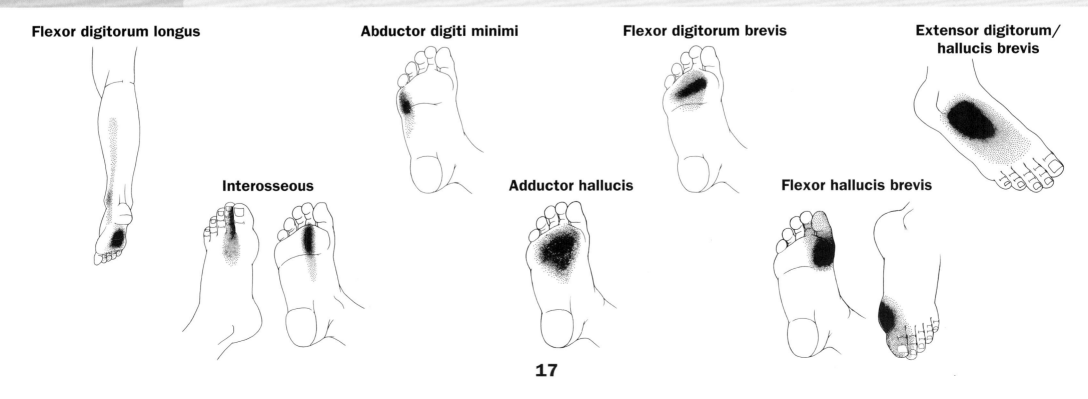

Flexor digitorum longus

Abductor digiti minimi

Flexor digitorum brevis

Extensor digitorum/hallucis brevis

Interosseous

Adductor hallucis

Flexor hallucis brevis

17